TABLE OF CONTENTS

Anti Aging Techniques EXPOSED Vol 5
Exercising to Prevent Aging
©Copyright 2013 by Dr. Noah Pranksky

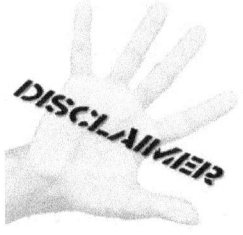

DISCLAIMER AND TERMS OF USE AGREEMENT:

(Please Read This Before Using This Book)

This information is for educational and informational purposes only. The content is not intended to be a substitute for any professional advice, diagnosis, or treatment.

The authors and publisher of this book and the accompanying materials have used their best efforts in preparing this book.

The authors and publisher make no representation or warranties with respect to the accuracy, applicability, fitness, or completeness of the contents of this book. The information contained in this book is strictly for educational purposes. Therefore, if you wish to apply ideas contained in this book, you are taking full responsibility for your actions.

The authors and publisher disclaim any warranties (express or implied), merchantability, or fitness for any particular purpose. The author and publisher shall in no event be held liable to any party for any direct, indirect, punitive, special, incidental or other consequential damages arising directly or indirectly from any use of this material, which is provided "as is", and without warranties. As always, the advice of a competent legal, tax, accounting, medical or other professional should be sought where applicable.

The authors and publisher do not warrant the performance, effectiveness or applicability of any sites listed or linked to in this book. All links are for information purposes only and are not warranted for content, accuracy or any other implied or explicit purpose. No part of this may be copied, or changed in any format, or used in any way other than what is outlined within this course under any circumstances. Violators will be prosecuted.

This book is © Copyrighted by ePubWealth.com.

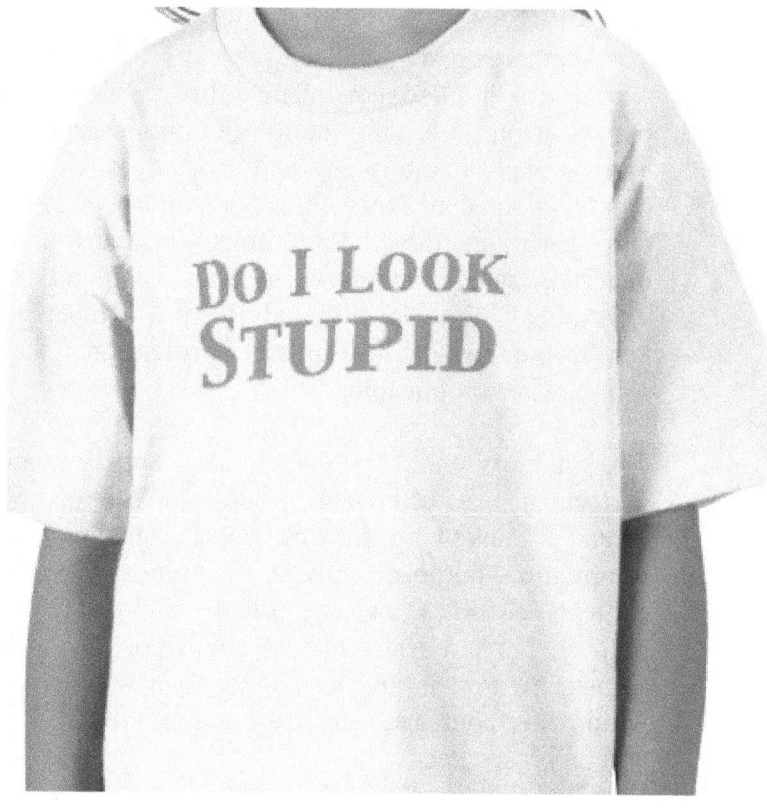

Although exercise is NOT a four-letter word, it does cause people to mutter certain expletives when the subject of exercise is brought up.

The psychology behind exercising is a type of reverse "cognitive dissonance". In science, cognitive dissonance is defined as "your actions being inconsistent with your beliefs".

4

In the case of exercising, reverse cognitive dissonance is defined as "your beliefs being inconsistence with your actions."

Everyone knows that exercising improves the quality of your life. This is a belief; however, because most people do not exercise, their beliefs are inconsistent with their actions.

When I refer to exercising, I am not referring to a consistent bodybuilding type of exercise program designed to put on muscle mass. In my opinion, bodybuilding is stupid because in most cases – not all – the human skeleton was not designed to hold the amount of muscle mass bodybuilders crave. It's like placing a skyscraper building on a residential home foundation. You would be utterly amazed at the statistics of how many bodybuilders require hip replacement and knee replacement surgeries after the age of 40.

What I am referring to is a daily consistent exercise routine that includes a light cardio workout and a light strength workout. Personally for my cardio workout I walk a minimum of 5-miles per day.

This gives me an added benefit of walking my dog and at the same time and giving him some play time to boot. It is a toss-up as to whether my dog prefers chasing the ball or chasing me.

For my strength workout, I follow along with an exercise video that uses light weights and isometric exercises. I want to feel good and look good but not for the sake of vanity and one of my most favorite sayings is, "Muscles get charley horses; baby fat NEVER gets a charley horse (lol)! That ought to be a bumper sticker!

So, we are going to "jump in" and begin by discussing just how much exercise a person needs. Men and women have different exercise needs and goal for that matter so we will also discuss this too.

And "NO," before you ask, you will not need a gallon jar of Ben-Gay. Remember, my take on exercise is the more sane and rational approach.
This is really going to shock you. Studies show that vigorous exercise offers virtually no additional mortality protection over moderate exercise. When your body has the optimal amount of EFAs, your endurance increases and exercise becomes easier.

A person burns 10-times as much glucose doing anaerobic exercise compared to the same amount of aerobic exercise.

It would take 10-hours of walking or 5-hours of aerobics to burn 1-pound of body fat.

A person eating 20% carbs/ 80% protein and natural fats after just 10-minutes of aerobics is burning 50% of energy from body fat. After 1-hour it is 65%!

To increase the release of HGH by the pituitary gland naturally there must be an increase in physical exercise, an increase in sleep plus the biochemical response to a HGH precursor formulation, which is widely available on the health market today. Release of HGH plus your low carb diet equals: increased lean muscle mass, increased strength, reduced body fat, steady anabolic rate and increased endurance.

Chapter 1 - Human Body Types

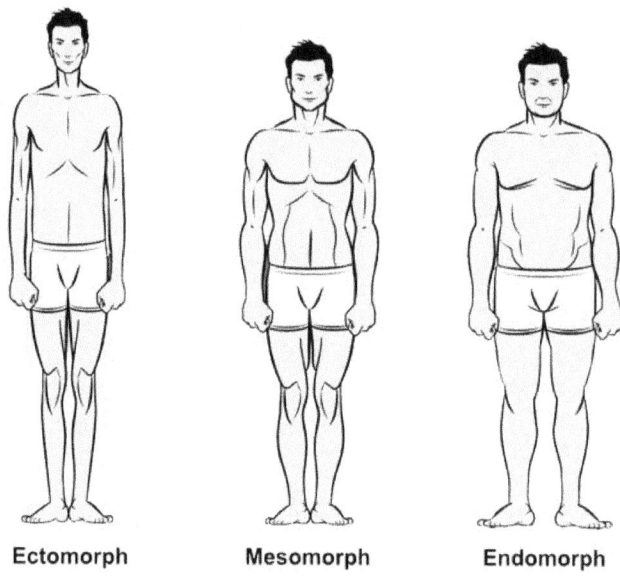

Ectomorph   Mesomorph   Endomorph

Endomorph

The Endomorph body type can build muscle successfully but will have to do so by using atypical methods. For example, the usual methods of bodybuilding do not work well for the Endomorph, due to his genetic propensity to store fat. "Work smarter, not harder" should be the motto of the Endomorph for he can get 100% faster and better results by understanding his own biochemistry.

Typical dieting and training will bring frustration to the Endomorph. He sees himself going by-the-book in diet and training, but just not getting the right results. The Endomorph is more psychologically tied to food, and to tell an Endomorph not to eat when he is hungry defies what his brain is telling him to do. The Endomorph will need to eat more low glycemic foods than any other body type as he will store fat very easily and will find it difficult to lose weight without starving.

Dropping calories will not work for the Endomorph, as the calories he craves, modifies his temperament. Instead of deprivation, the Endomorph should eat when he is hungry - just eat the right foods. No high or moderately high glycemic foods; i.e., sucrose, bananas, or raisins as they exacerbate the Endomorph's fat storing tendencies. Aerobic exercise will be the key factor for the Endomorph bodybuilder. He will have to run, bike; take aerobics, etc. to hold a very low body fat level. Swimming should be avoided by the Endomorph, as it will add body fat (unless the Endomorph is a very heavy swimmer).

The Endomorph endurance athlete won't have a problem with extra body fat until he stops training. The Endomorph bodybuilder, or strength athlete, will achieve success by following a regimen of high-sets and high-reps combined with 30-minutes of aerobic exercise every day and a very low glycemic diet of no less than 1,800 calories per day.

Mesomorph

The Mesomorph is the most muscular of all the Somatotypes. He naturally has some muscle whether he exercises or not. The typical Mesomorph has a thick muscle structure, a large chest, thick arms and legs, and is extremely strong.

The Mesomorph can build muscle easily and with the right diet can become massive as well as ripped. The key for the Mesomorph body type in bodybuilding is diet. He possesses all the physical basics, so it is just a matter of chiseling down the sculpture to the proper dimensions. The Mesomorph can easily hold too much water, and needs to move that water into the muscle and out of the subcutaneous fat so he looks large and defined.

He can only accomplish this through diet and not by any exercise or weightlifting program alone. Obviously an excellent weight-training program is essential, but to the Mesomorph, diet is number one! He has already been blessed genetically, which makes his muscles respond quickly to training.

The Mesomorph must eat more protein than the other two body types. His ancestors, Australopithecus Africanus, were hunters and gatherers, and as such, consumed as much live protein as they could catch. Trying to change thousands of years of genetic programming is a waste of time.

The bodybuilding Mesomorph needs to maintain his constant weight (within 10 lbs.) year round. He needs to eat 30 to 50 grams of high quality, lean protein as food and/or acceptable weight gain powders, 5-6 times a day. Ingesting more than around 50 grams of protein at one time is counter-productive and will not result in more lean muscle mass.

A Mesomorph should not attempt to hold the same body fat level as an ectomorph. The latest data reflects that in many Mesomorphs, ingesting less than 30% fat in their diet results in the Mesomorph muscle "flattening out". This means manipulating the type of fats in the Mesomorph diet is much more important than simply reducing the total fat intake to the typically recommended 15% to 20%. The high oleic monounsaturated fats should replace the polyunsaturated and saturated fats.

The Mesomorph bodybuilder should consume 1 gram of lean protein for every pound of lean muscle mass (not total weight). This should be eaten with cruciferous vegetables (for proper metabolism of protein) and low to moderate glycemic carbs for a total daily intake of not less than 2200 balanced calories.

Ectomorph

The Ectomorph will need to take in more calories than most body types, as their metabolism is so efficient it burns up food easily and effectively. They usually have to eat consistently to gain weight, and may be underweight. Properly formulated weight gain powders are usually required to add muscle mass to the Ectomorph.

What the ectomorph does not need is sucrose or glucose in foods, supplements or weight gainers as those types of sugars tend to make his abdominal region round and soft. Ectomorphs are usually extremely flexible. They also make excellent long distance runners. In training, an Ectomorph will need to work harder to build maximum

11

muscle, and will need a lot of sleep (8-10 hours per night).

If they are not gaining muscle, then caloric and total nutrient intake will need to increase and they will need to eat more frequently. Unlike the other body types, the Ectomorph can usually eat as much food as he desires and not gain weight. That same metabolic blessing becomes a problem when attempting to add muscle mass.

An Ectomorph can usually eat more high glycemic foods than the other two body types and not gain body fat. If an Ectomorph is gaining too much body fat as they work to gain muscle, they can eat foods lower in the glycemic index. For an Ectomorph, they key to gaining muscle mass is to steadily increase their total daily intake of calories until muscle mass is evidenced.

Ectomorphs have been known to consume from 8,000 to 10,000 calories per day before gaining substantial muscle mass. In bodybuilding Ectomorphs, very intense weight training balanced with long rest periods is essential. Aerobic exercise should be kept to a minimum, as an Ectomorph who gets a lot of aerobic exercise can easily develop a body profile of 98% lean mass with 2% body fat.

The Ectomorph will feel lethargic if he does not get exercise of some type at least three times per week. For cardiovascular fitness, using the Stairmaster or swimming for 1/2 hour, three times per week, would suit the Ectomorph's system.

Chapter 2 - Preparation Stage - How Much Exercise Do You Need?

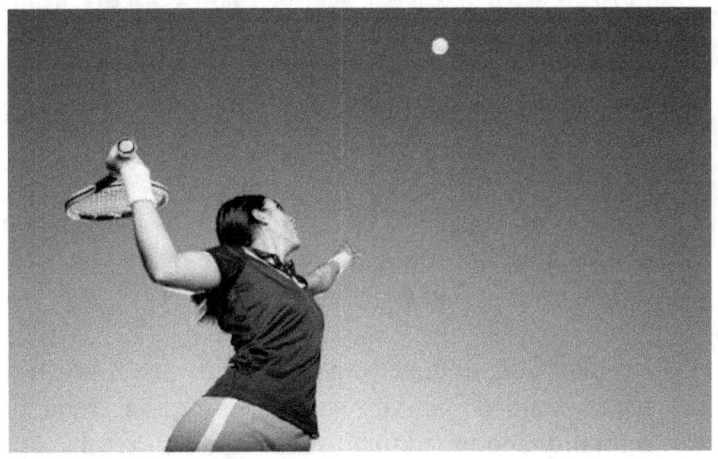

If you listen to all the hype regarding exercises, it seems like everyone has a different take on how much exercise you need: 1 hour, 3 times a week; 30 minutes a day; so much aerobic, strength, flexibility, etc. These recommendations are based on a combination of science, common sense and "best guess." What happens when you look at a large group of people over a long time and see how the people who followed the guidelines did in terms of longevity and life expectancy?

In a giant survey of 252,925 men and women aged 50 to 71 years, researchers examined reported physical activity levels (compared those to current recommendations) and looked at health outcomes. Over the course of the study, 7,900 participants died. Researchers compared those that died to the rest to determine the impact of exercise. Here is what they found:

People who exercised moderately at least 30 minutes most days of the week were 27% less likely to die over the course of the study.

People who exercised vigorously at least 20 minutes, three times a week were 32% less likely to die.

This benefit existed even in sub-groups like smokers, the overweight, the obese, and people who watched more than 2 hours a day of television.

People who engaged in less than the two levels of recommended activity also showed a reduction in mortality compared to those that did no exercise.

Exercise is Good For You

Exercise is good and will help you live longer and it makes you feel good as long as you don't over or under do it. The current recommendations seem accurate; you should try to either exercise moderately for 30 minutes most days or vigorously for 20 minutes at least three times a week.

Jump Start Your Exercise

Use the tips offered in this volume and ideas to inspire your exercise motivation and get back into a strong weekly exercise plan. Exercise is one of the best ways to add years to your life and tap into the hidden quality of life benefits of exercise.

Buy New Exercise Clothes

A lot of people are motivated by clothes. If you happen to be one of them, go for it. Buy that new workout outfit, get the new shoes, invest in some nice things. The more you spend, the more likely you will be to use those clothes. It's just human nature.

So give yourself a budget and renew your passion for exercise through your passion for new clothes.

Get a New Exercise Video

Exercise videos are great - you get some of the benefits of a group class without having to leave your house and I swear by them because I can follow along and stay focused. There's an instructor to demonstrate the proper form and give tips, and (most importantly) to keep track of time. If you need to rev up your workout, go shopping and find some new exercise videos. Pick ones that look fun and work on mastering those workouts. When they get sale, buy some new ones. It's a lot cheaper than a gym membership.

Morning Exercise to Start Your Day Right

I do my walking and exercises in the morning when I have the most energy and it is cool. It also helps to rev up my metabolism all day long. Not only will you feel more energy, you also might sleep better. Most importantly, by exercising in the morning you'll be sure to get your workout in every single day before interruptions and distractions start up.

Find the Best Exercise Music

For me, it is my iPod that gets me out exercising. A new album can have me looking forward to a run like nothing else. Not only does music get me out exercising more, it also helps increase the intensity of my workouts. You can get a cheap music player and load it up -- it can transform exercise from a chore to something exciting.

Chapter 3 - Equipment - Exercise Bikes, Treadmills and Rowing Machines

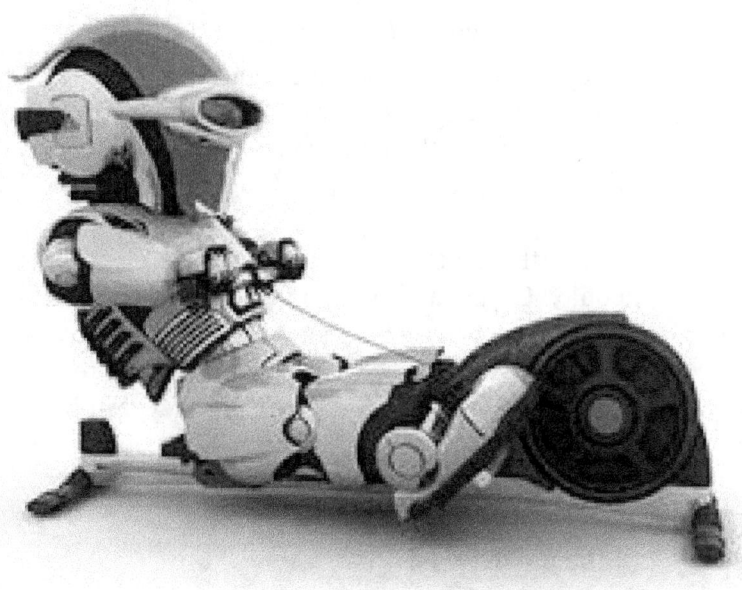

Home exercise equipment (bikes, treadmills and rowing machines) can offer excellent workouts and provide necessary aerobic exercise. The trick is to figure out how to transform using them from being a dreadful chore to being something to look forward to.

I like to use any "machine exercise" time to do something I don't usually have time for: read a book. In my case, I listen to a book. I'll go online and download that latest book that just looks great and hit "play" while I sweat on the machine. If I had a handy TV nearby, I might rent some movies I've been wanting to see. The key is to find something exciting so that, on a bad day, you still want to exercise so you can finish the movie or book or whatever else motivates you.

Group Exercise = Better Effort

Group exercise classes are fantastic. Not only do you benefit from an instructor pushing you for the entire hour or so, you also benefit from someone else setting your exercise schedule for you.

To get the most out of a group exercise class, talk to people. Come a few minutes early and chat with the instructor or other classmates. Be sure to tell people at the end of class, "See you next time." The more interactions you have, the more social pressure they will be for you to return. In this case, peer pressure is a good thing that will keep you exercising on a low motivation day.

Make an Exercise Plan

Make a plan for yourself, set some goals, become determined. Get a big calendar and circle the days you want to exercise. Put a big "X" through them when you do. Give yourself a reward for a perfect week and a perfect month. Make no compromises or excuses - stick with your plan.

Exercise Mats for Home Workouts

When people think of working out at home, they usually think of some kind of machine -- an exercise bike, rowing machine or treadmill. These can, of course, be great. My favorite home exercise piece of equipment is a simple exercise mat (or yoga mat). This is just something you unroll on the floor to allow yourself a padded space to stretch and do strengthening using your body weight. An exercise mat and a couple of videos is all you need to get started. You'd be surprised just how good of a workout you can get with simple equipment.

Have a Ball with an Exercise Ball

If you are just getting started exercising and don't want to make a big investment, consider an exercise ball. They are inexpensive, can be used at home and will really open up possibilities for your workout. Find an exercise ball that comes with a video to help you learn some of the exercises you can do. You may need to buy some light weights to do with it -- but that's it. An exercise ball could be all you need for a great workout.

Top Anti-Aging and Exercise Articles

Lots of exercise recommendations are out there. While many are good, most are designed to help athletes reach peak performance or to help people lose weight.

When it comes to exercising for longevity, things get a bit muddy. Is it better to focus on your heart, bones or muscles? Is there an age when the risks of exercise outweigh the benefits? These articles look into some research and other ideas to help you exercise for a longer life.

Walk Away Metabolic Syndrome

Metabolic syndrome is a fancy name that means someone is headed for lots of trouble. The typical person with metabolic syndrome is overweight, has high cholesterol and a host of other problems. A person with metabolic syndrome is at high risk for heart disease and diabetes.

The good news is that taking control of your lifestyle can really help. One change that helps -- walking. Getting a bit of daily walking can derail metabolic syndrome and put a person on a path toward greater health.

Chapter 4 - Exercise, Life Expectancy and Longevity

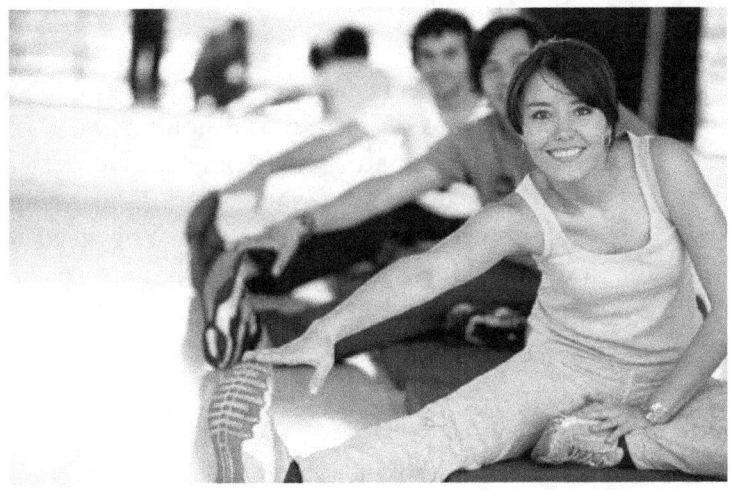

We're not just about living longer, we want to live longer AND feel good doing. A 65-year-old who exercises regularly can expect to live without any disabilities until 83 (add in a healthy diet and that number can increase even more). So live long and live well by exercising.

Hidden Benefits of Exercise

You probably already know that exercise is good for your heart and can help keep the weight off -- but did you know it was good for sex? How about mood? Sleep? There are tons of benefits of exercise that go way beyond longevity and staying healthy.

Exercise will help you feel great today and every day. So start exercising and pay attention to these hidden benefits to keep yourself motivated.

Make Exercise Fun

So you're convinced that exercise is a good thing and you know you need to do it at least 3 hours a week. Now is the most important part -- find some way to get yourself excited about exercise. Anything you are planning to do for 3 hours a week needs to be fun. You need to look forward to exercise. Sit down and brainstorm ways to work up a sweat and have a good time doing so. These ideas can help.

Learn to Love Exercise

If you are a true beginner to exercise, it is going to take a while to make exercise a habit. You are going to need to start small and build up strength and endurance. Forget everything you read (except this, of course) and what people tell you. The most important thing is to work on building exercise into your weekly routine. If you can do that, everything else will follow. Set aside time for exercise and physical activity and don't let anything stand in your way. After a month or two, you'll be loving exercise (really, you will -- just give it a try).

Boost the Benefit - Add 14 More Years

Exercise is good, but if you can combine it with a few other behaviors you can really boost the benefit. People, who don't smoke, eat 5 servings of fruits and vegetables and have 1 to 2 drinks of alcohol a day live 14 years longer than people who don't do those things. An after work-out banana, a double serving of vegetables and a glass of wine. These are simple pleasures that are healthy and anti-aging.

Your Brain on Exercise - for the 85+ Crowd

At 85, you may think that you have no need to start exercise -- this is wrong. Not only will exercise help with balance and flexibility, it will actually help keep your brain healthy. So if you (or your parents) are in the 85-ish crowd, be sure to keep on exercising. Your brain will be happier, healthier and younger.

Stroke Risk and Physical Activity

Speaking of brains, a stroke is one of the most debilitating and life threatening things that can happen. In a stroke, the blood vessels rupture in the brain and cause damage such as lose of the ability to speak and problems moving. Prevent strokes by watching your blood pressure and keeping your blood vessels healthy through (you guessed it) exercise.

Lifestyle Changes Benefit Middle Aged

I've talked to a lot of people in their 50s and 60s who think there is no point in starting a healthy lifestyle now. They are overweight and have unhealthy diets. They think the damage is done. The "why bother" attitude is dead wrong.

Making lifestyle changes in a person's middle ages can have tremendous benefit. Give these changes a month and see if you don't start feeling better. Focus on the immediate benefits like better sleep, more energy and an improved mood.

Make Your DNA Younger

With over 1,200 pairs of twins enrolled in the study, researchers were able to determine the impact of exercise on the telomere length of white blood cells. In short, they could measure how exercise can make DNA younger and healthier.

This is a huge new step in understanding how lifestyle plays a role in aging.

What Exercise is Good For DNA?

Working up a sweat seems to be important. People who exercised vigorously at least 3 hours each week had longer telomeres and were 9 years younger than couch potatoes who did no exercise.

This holds true after removing other factors like smoking, age, weight and activity level at work.

So What If My Telomeres Are Short?

Researchers believe that shortened telomeres can increase the risk of age-related diseases like high blood pressure, mental difficulties, cancer and more.

This is because as telomeres shorten, there is more stress on your body's tissues to function correctly.

Researchers believe that exercise helps reduce damage by free radicals, allowing your body to invest its resources in maintaining health instead of repairing damage.

Conclusion
Exercise three hours a day not just for your DNA, but also to feel good and experience all the benefits of exercise.

Chapter 5 - Do It for the Right Reason - Exercise for a Long Life

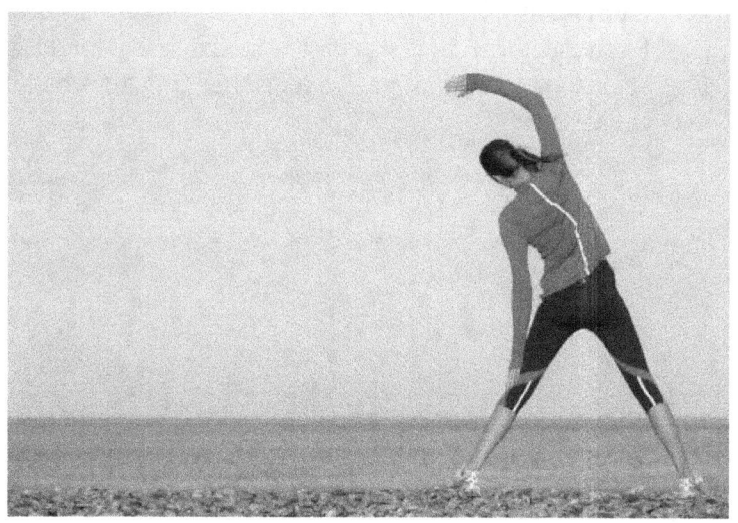

Exercise is one of the most important things you can do. Without exercise, you increase your risk of a wide assortment of chronic illnesses. Here is a list of conditions that physical activity can reduce the risk for (and how many people have them):

- Coronary Heart Disease (12.6 million)
- Heart Attack (1.1 million)
- Diabetes (17 million)
- Hip Fracture (300,000)
- High Blood Pressure (50 million)
- Obesity (50 million)
- Overweight (108 million)

Exercise Adds Years to Your Life

One study found that the average 65-year-old can expect an additional 12.7 years of healthy life –- meaning he will live disability-free until age 77.7. Highly active 65-years-olds, however, have an additional 5.7 years of healthy life expectancy –- they will remain disability free until age 83.4.

Another study found that increasing physical activity after age 50 can add years to one's life. In the study, individuals with and without cardiovascular disease were compared by the amount of physical activity they did.

Men who were moderately active added 1.3 years to their lives and those who were highly active added 3.7 years.

Women who were moderately active added 1.1 years and those were highly active added 3.2 years. In addition, people who exercised more also lived more years free of cardiovascular disease.

While moderate exercise increases life expectancy, highly active people more than doubled the benefits.

Get Started

Get started exercising by increasing your physical activity every day. Walk more, get up more and just use your body. Then add in 30-minute periods that you commit to exercise. Do some strength, balance and stretching work. Find a time every day and commit to doing something that's physical.

Hidden Benefits of Exercise

Everyone knows that exercise is good for your heart and helps you stay slimmer, but did you know that exercise also improves your balance? Helps you sleep better at night? Puts you in a good mood? Learn more about the hidden benefits of exercise to help motivate your exercise habits.

Energize With Exercise

Routine exercise will increase your energy level. Exercise will make you feel great and you'll be able to take on more than you ever thought possible. Regular exercise also decreases your chance of developing fatigue and exhaustion. So instead of feeling run down, go for a run.

Want Better Sex? Exercise More

Better sex has been linked to higher levels of physical activity. The more you exercise, the better your circulation and the more sensitive you are to sexual pleasure. Frequent exercise will also help your body image, allowing you to relax more during sex.

Allow me to add one very important ingredient into the mix of sex. This will seem more like common sense but you would be surprised at how often I am asked this question. Sex is NOT a requirement of the human body. No one has ever died due to the lack of sex. In fact, in times of famine or severe dieting, the body will shut down all unnecessary functions to divert nutrients to the organs.

Yep, SEX is the first thing to go so remember, the optimum sex occurs along with optimum health.

Exercise Improves Sleep

Exercise, especially morning exercise, can improve your sleep quality. Researchers believe that morning exercise helps to set your body clock each day. This in turn makes you feel awake during the day and tired at night. Try some morning exercise for a week and see if your sleep improves.

Chapter 6 - The Exercise / Sleep Connection

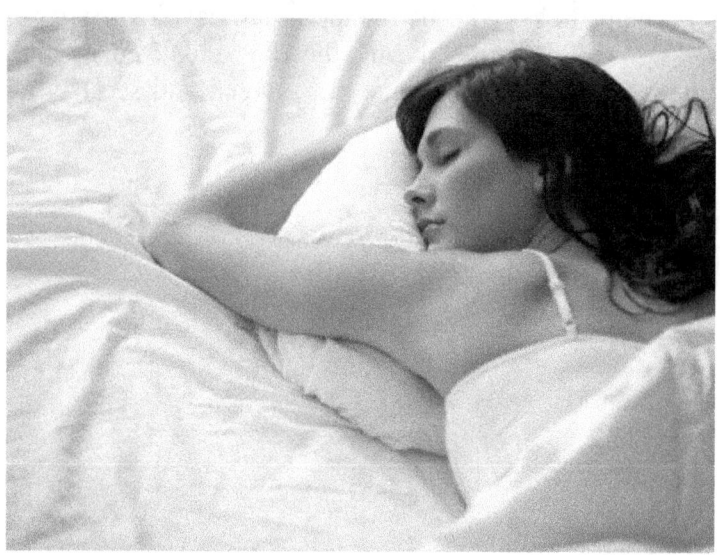

Keep Your Brain Sharp by Exercising Your Body

If you though Sudoku was a great brain workout, try playing tennis. Physical activity requires a lot of participation from our brain. In exercise, you must make quick decisions, judgment calls, find the best strategies. People who remain physical active as they age have a reduced risk of dementia and cognitive decline.

Exercise, Brain Health and Aging
Exercise and Be Happy

When you exercise, your body releases chemicals that make you feel good. These chemicals can improve your body and help you relax. Exercise also makes you feel good about yourself. It can improve your mood and even help ease the symptoms of mild to moderate depression.

Exercise Adds Years to Your Life

Not only does exercise add years to your life, it also increases the number of years that you live without disease or disability. If you are 65, adding in exercise now can add over 5 additional years of disability free living (on average). If you are younger than 65, the benefits can be even greater.

Fight Colds with Exercise

Exercise improves your immune system. People who are physically active are less likely to catch a cold. And if you have a mild cold, a little bit of exercise can help speed your recovery. So increase the power of your immune system by going for a walk, joining the gym or dusting off your bike and going for a ride.

Exercise Your Bones

Your bones need stimulation to stay strong. Weight bearing exercises help increase your bone density and strength. Be sure to include exercises like running or walking that put weight one your bones. And don't forget to add in some resistance and weight training too.

Exercise Improves Balance

Regular exercise can improve your sense of balance. This is especially important as you age. Lack of balance can lead to falls and hip fractures. Follow these simple instructions for balance exercises that you can do at home. Research has shown that exercises like these will reduce your risk of falling.

Be Social - Exercise

Exercise is a great way to meet people and be more social. There are plenty of group exercise activities that you can do that will give you both physical and social benefits. Be sure to work at least one social exercise routine into your week - both your physical and social health will improve.

Make Exercise Fun (How To)

Exercise is one of the pillars of longevity. The benefits of exercise are many: heart health, weight management, better sleep, improved mood, more energy and many more. The biggest benefit? Reducing your risk of chronic illnesses. Through exercise, you'll stay healthy longer, age well and feel great.

Getting started on a routine exercise habit is the hardest part. Use these 10 ways to put some more fun into your exercise routine.

1. **Add a Friend**

    Find someone to be your exercise buddy. Don't choose just anyone: Pick someone who is full of energy, fun and who you look forward to spending time with. That way, you'll want to exercise just to be with your friend.

2. **Group Fitness**

Group classes are a way to meet new people, have an instructor to keep your form and effort good and be motivated to go each time. Shop around for your class: Find an instructor who has both knowledge and enthusiasm. You can gauge the social tone an instructor creates by watching if anyone talks to him or her before or after the class and if the other participants talks to each other.

3. Play Something

We use the word "play" in front of sports because they are fun. You "play" tennis, golf, soccer, softball or any other sport. Find a sport that you used to "play" when younger and take it up again. Choose a team sport when possible to add some socialization.

4. Audio Books and Podcasts

Get yourself a tiny music player and download some audio books or podcasts. Hundreds of free podcasts are available covering any topic you can imagine. Audio books can also be easily downloaded. This way, when you think about exercising, you can be looking forward to "reading" the next chapter in your novel.

5. New Shoes

Go exercise-fashion shopping. Start with your shoes. Go to a good running or fitness store and have a salesperson help you find the perfect shoe.

Each type of shoe supports you foot differently, so you need to make sure you have the right shoe for you. Bring in your old running or exercise shoes; the wear marks will tell the salesperson how you run. After the luster wears off your shoes, go back for some new shorts, shirts or other accessories.

6. Chart Your Stats

Thousands of people obsessively chart the stats of their favorite baseball, basketball or football players and teams. Do the same for yourself. Create a wall chart and log your exercise activity, vital statistics (weight, measurements, best times, maximum lifts, etc.). Chart every detail of your exercise routine for a month. You'll feel great as the information gets up on the wall.

7. Mix It Up

Don't do the exact same exercise routine every day; mix it up. If you always run on the treadmill, run outside on a nice day. Take a week off your lifting routine and do a Pilates class instead. As soon as you feel your exercise routine becoming a rut, find something else to do.

8. Measure, Don't Weigh

The scale can be the worst factor when it comes to motivation. You may be working hard, but your weight just stays the same. Part of the reason may be that you are adding muscle while losing fat. Another reason is that it just takes time and changes in your diet to lose substantial weight. So stop looking at the scale every day; instead, take some measurements. The tape measure will show change well before the scale does. Measure your chest, upper arms, stomach, waist, upper thighs and calves. Be sure to measure in the same place each time. Add those measurements to your wall chart and watch the progress.

9. TV, Videos and Music

Many people find that a bit of distraction helps get them through a workout. Get a tiny music player and load it up with inspirational music (change the music weekly to give you some surprises). Watch TV shows while on the treadmill or put in your favorite movie and watch 1/2 of it each time you exercise. That way, you'll be able to watch one or two movies a week. You can do the same with TV shows; record your shows or rent a series and watch while exercising. You'll look forward to your exercise just to find out what happens next in the show.

10. Relax

At the end of exercise (after you "cool down"), give yourself 5 minutes of relaxation. Just lie down on your back and let your body sink into the floor. Close your eyes. Relax. Feel the effects of exercise in your body. Look forward to the deep relaxation that can come after physical activity. You may find that you start exercising just to experience this feeling.

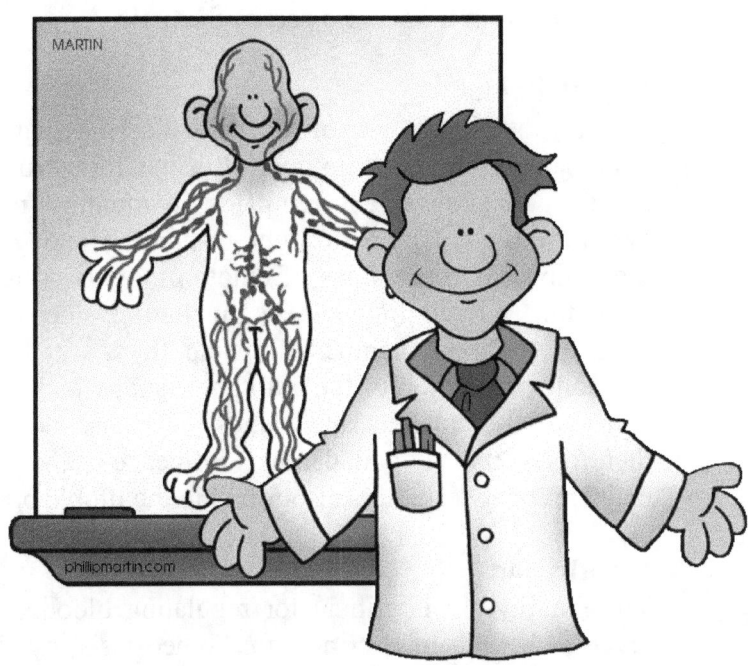

Please be advised that I have to make a legal disclaimer now: I do not endorse/ recommend, suggest or promote any of the products, devices, and or protocols on any of the pages contained herein. Nor do I suggest that you avoid a medical practitioner for any reason. I make no claim whether implied or written
The Endocrine System

Pineal

The function of the Pineal is not well understood; this gland has been referred to as the "third eye." Its only major secretion is melatonin, which influences sleep cycles. It is strongly influenced by cycles of daylight, and is found in the limbric part of the brain.

Hypothalamus
The Hypothalamus is not a true endocrine gland; the hypothalamus is the main control center for virtually all organs and tissues. It regulates involuntary nervous system activity (flight or fight responses) and governs most physical expressions of emotions. It is critical for regulating overall homeostasis, including sleep cycles, food intake, body temperature, and thirst. It controls hormone production of the pituitary gland, which in turn, stimulates other endocrine glands to release hormones; therefore, the hypothalamus influences the entire endocrine network. It is also found in the limbic brain.

Parathyroid
The Parathyroid is critical for regulating blood calcium levels (which itself is critical for homeostasis) by pulling calcium from the bones and reabsorbing it through the kidneys. It also contributes to phosphorus and vitamin D metabolism. It is on the thyroid gland.

Pituitary
The Pituitary, about the size of a pea, is considered the "master gland" because many of its secretions regulate hormone production in the other endocrine glands. Its own hormones affect cell growth, protein synthesis, glucose utilization, fat metabolism, and the regulation of

most chemical reactions in general. Found in the limbic brain.

Thyroid
The Thyroid is the body's major regulator of metabolic activity, primarily through the oxidation of glucose and oxygen consumption. It helps regulate food and calcium metabolism, body temperature, tissue, bone and nervous system development, and is essential for the development and regulation of the female reproductive system. It also affects protein synthesis, heart function, blood pressure and respiration. It is found in the neck.

Adrenal
The Adrenal is found on top of the kidneys, the adrenals function as two separate glands. They utilize cholesterol to synthesize dozens of steroid hormones that help regulate fluid electrolyte balances (especially sodium), affect sex drive, stimulate the body into "flight or fight" action, and at the same time maintain a state of "crisis management". In terms of sheer stress response, the adrenal glands are the star players.

Thymus
The Thymus is considered essential for the normal development of the immune response. It activates lymphocytes to recognize specific pathogens. It is located behind the breast bone.

Ovary
The Ovary produces estrogens and progesterone, which affect all aspects of the development of sexual activity. They also help regulate cholesterol levels and calcium.

Testes

The testes are a gland that produces the male reproductive cells and the male hormone testosterone.

Prostaglandin

Prostaglandin is considered to be "local" hormones, found in virtually all cell membranes. There many functions include hormone regulation, gastric secretion, platelet aggregation, and inflammation responses.

Uterus

The uterus contains and nourishes the embryo and fetus, and aids in balancing hormones.

Prostate

The prostate is partly glandular and partly muscular. The gland secretes a thin opalescent, slightly alkaline fluid that forms part of the semen.

The Digestive System

Digestive System

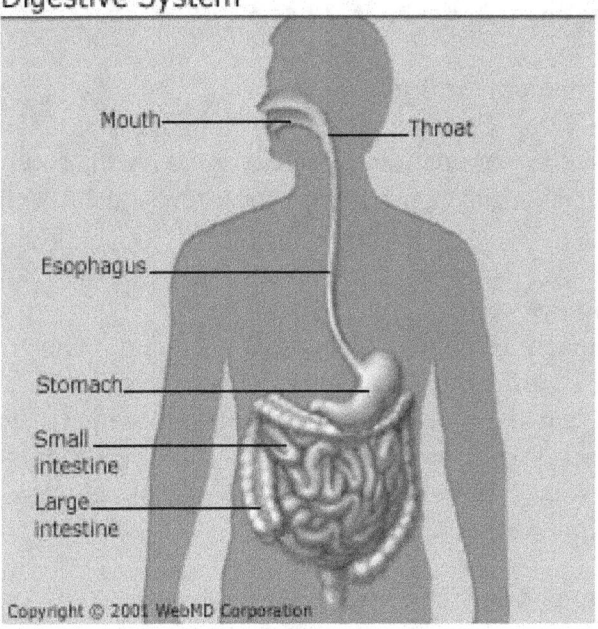

Mouth — Throat

Esophagus

Stomach

Small intestine

Large intestine

Copyright © 2001 WebMD Corporation

The digestive system is much more than just a place to put the things we eat. It is a complex refinery that converts foodstuffs into the majority of the nutritional tools we need to maintain health and wellness. If these are not viable options – if any part of the food processing operation becomes compromised through injury, substance abuse, or poor dietary habits – then the digestive system becomes a pathway to potential toxicity.

Parotid Gland
The Parotid Gland is a large salivary gland near the ear, stimulated to produce saliva by the presence of food in the mouth. Saliva contains certain antibodies and

enzymes that play a major role in preventing pathogens from entering the body.

Temporomandibular Joint
The Temporomandibular Joint facilitates chewing, which, with the stimulation of saliva mixed with food, is the most significant process in the prevention of absorbing parasites.

Stomach Acid
Stomach Acid contains hydrochloric acid, which not only is a significant pathogenic inhibitor; it is also required to activate the stomach enzyme pepsin, which begins the breakdown of proteins for further processing in the small intestine. Without pepsin, proteins can begin to putrefy in the stomach.

Gallbladder
The Gallbladder is a "way" station for liver bile and can accumulate toxins, especially those of synthetic chemical origins.

Intrinsic Factor
Intrinsic Factor is produced only n the stomach and is a substance required for the absorption of B-12 in the small intestine.

Liver
The Liver is the primary site for the enzymatic breakdown of toxins and their subsequent removal via the kidneys and intestines.

Pancreas

The Pancreas produces most of the protease, lipase, and amylase (all digestive enzymes) involved in digestion, as well as juices that neutralize stomach acid in the small intestine.

Small Intestine
The Small Intestine is the recipient of all foods and digestive juices and its function can be affected by any imbalances in the stomach, pancreas, liver and / or gallbladder.

Valve Houston
The Valve Houston is one of the mucosal folds of the rectum, and plays a role in controlling intestinal parasites.

Large Intestines
The Large Intestines reabsorb water from undigested materials and eliminates the consolidated waste. The "friendly" bacteria of the gut provide some digestion, but mostly contribute to controlling the growth and spread of harmful bacteria, and to the production of some B-complex vitamins and vitamin K.

Bowl Flora
Bowl Flora provides the best defense against invading harmful bacteria in the gut.

Ileocecal Valve
The Ileocecal Valve prevents fecal material from backing up into the small intestine.

Micelle Balance

Micelles are micro-clusters of fat-based molecules that transport nutrients through the small intestine. Bioenergetically, micelle balance represents the body's capacity to absorb and regulate the distribution of nutrients.

The Immune System

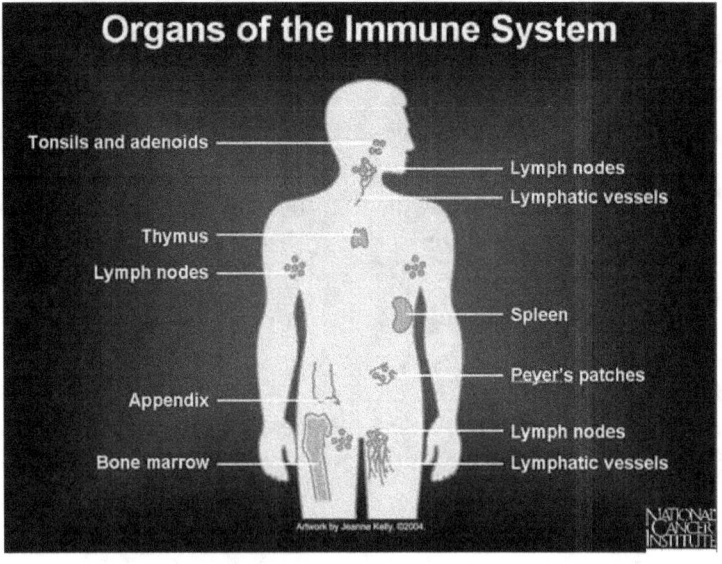

Detoxification itself is a defensive measure, but it is assisted greatly by the immune system proper. The immune system might be considered the border guard of our protective network. A healthy immune system is critical to the balanced body.

This does not mean an immune system that is constantly stimulated, but rather one that is fully functional, conserving its resources and ready to do battle when necessary. "Necessary" results from injury, invasion or imbalance.

The first two are usually temporary responses, but the imbalance can trigger the immune system for the long haul.

Lymphatic
The Lymphatic System is our first line of internal defense; a vast network of drainage ducts and glands designed to remove wastes, toxins and pathogens from the blood via a plasma-like fluid called lymph. The lymphatic network is also critical to supporting the cardiovascular system by returning leaked fluids to the bloodstream.

Brain
Our thought processes have direct impacts on the chemicals released by the brain, which in turn stimulate the autonomic (involuntary) nervous system to respond to incoming and perceived stressors.

Thymus
The Thymus produces specific lymphocytes to attack viruses, bacteria and abnormal cell growths.

Tonsils / Adenoids

The Tonsils / Adenoids are sites of concentrated lymph tissue for trapping and destroying bacteria entering the body through ingestion or inhalation.

Liver
The Liver is the primary site for the enzymatic breakdown of toxins and their subsequent removal via the kidneys and intestines.

Skin
The Skin is the largest detoxifying organ of the body, and is capable of exerting as many toxins as the kidneys through its oil glands and sweat pores. The Skin is our first line of external defense.

Appendix
The Appendix is a major lymphoid organ, ideally situated for processing the bacteria of the large intestine.

Bowl Flora
Bowl Flora provides the best defense against invading harmful bacteria in the gut.

Bone Marrow
Bone Marrow is the site of red blood cell and lymphocyte (white blood cell) production.

Connective Tissue
Connective Tissue is the most abundant and widespread tissue in the body. Home to the meridian system, it is the primary communication network of the body in terms of the bionetic information that serves to maintain homeostasis and health.

It becomes the depository for many of the toxins that are not completely metabolized or eliminated through the normal processes of detoxification.

The Lymphatic System

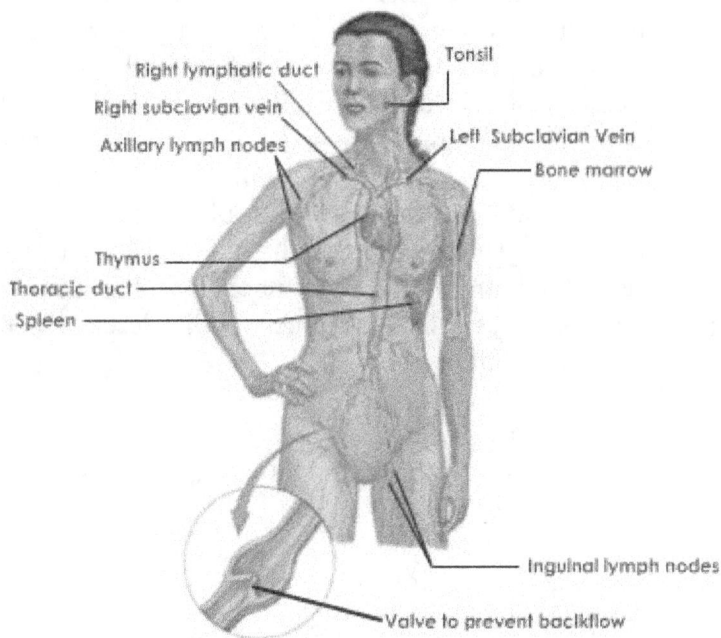

The massive network of the lymphatic system is our first line of internal defense. Twice as extensive as the circulatory system, it removes pathogens and waste products from the bloodstream and sends them through a series of vessels that occasionally expand into areas of concentrated lymphoid tissue called "node", where the pathogens are destroyed by lymphocytes and macrophages. The cleansed lymph is then returned to the bloodstream through the subclavian veins. The fluid known as "lymph" does not move actively through the system, but relies on the physical action of the skeletal muscles and diaphragm for transport. Even so, the lymph movement is slow and uneven, emphasizing the grave importance of physical activity in maintaining overall health. Another critical factor to health is the lymph's role in returning interstitial and plasma proteins to the bloodstream. This fluid is forced out of the blood when it moves from the arterial capillaries to venous capillaries. Although the amount is relatively small – about three liters per day – this fluid must be returned to the bloodstream for the cardiovascular system to function properly. Thus, if the lymphatic is to serve us, we must serve the lymph! Since the function of the various lymph vessels is basically the same, we will describe here only the areas of drainage.

Subclavian (Trunks)
The Subclavian Trunks drains the upper arms.

Cervical (Nodes)
Cervical Nodes are located near the cervical vertebrae, servicing the head and trunk.

Lymphoreticular (Tissue)

Lymphoreticular Tissue is pertaining to the mesh-like network of cells that forms the lining of the lymphatic vessels.

Axillary (Nodes)
Axillary Nodes are found in the chest near the armpits.

Right Nymphatic (Duct)
The Right Nymphatic Duct drains the right arm and the right side of the head and thorax.

Thoracic (Duct)
The Thoracic Duct drains the rest of the body.

Abdominal (Nodes)
The Abdominal Nodes are found throughout the abdomen, but mainly clustered around the abdominal aorta.

Cysterna Chyli
The Cysterna Chyli is an enlarged sac of the thoracic duct that collects lymph from the legs and abdomen.

Inguinal (Nodes)
The Inguinal Nodes are located in the groin area.

Peripheral (Nodes)
The Peripheral Nodes are scattered throughout the connective tissue in the outlying areas of the body.

I Have a Special Gift for My Readers

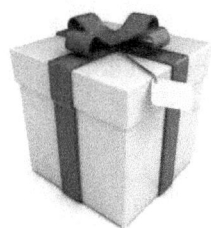

I appreciate my readers for without them I am just another author attempting to make a difference. If my book has made a favorable impression please leave me an honest review. Thank you in advance for you participation.

My readers and I have in common a passion for the written word as well as the desire to learn and grow from books.

My special offer to you is a massive ebook library that I have compiled over the years. It contains hundreds of fiction and non-fiction ebooks in Adobe Acrobat PDF format as well as the Greek classics and old literary classics too.

In fact, this library is so massive to completely download the entire library will require over 5 GBs open on your desktop.

Use the link below and scan all of the ebooks in the library. You can select the ebooks you want individually or download the entire library.

The link below does not expire after a given time period so you are free to return for more books rather than clog your desktop. And feel free to give the link to your friends who enjoy reading too.

I thank you for reading my book and hope if you are pleased that you will leave me an honest review so that I can improve my work and or write books that appeal to your interests.

Okay, here is the link…

http://tinyurl.com/special-readers-promo

PS: If you wish to reach me personally for any reason you may simply write to mailto:support@epubwealth.com.

I answer all of my emails so rest assured I will respond.

Meet the Author

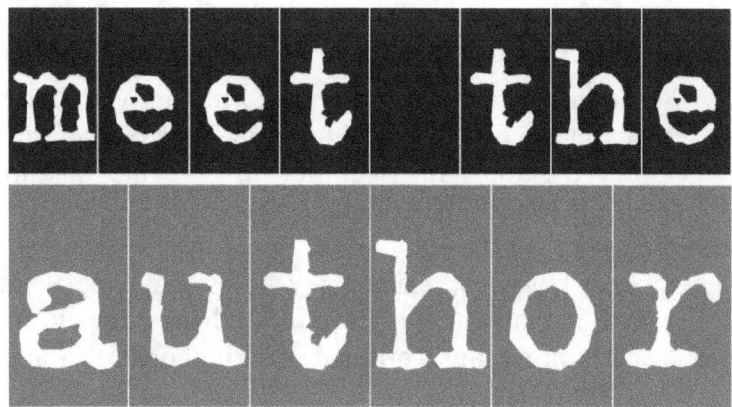

Dr. Noah Pranksky is a research behavioral scientist for Applied Mind Sciences. His research involves many aspects of the human mind including relationships, energy psychology, and various protocols and modalities relating to treatment and cure of various mental maladies.

He and his wife Marianne reside in Portland, Oregon.

Visit some of his websites
http://www.AddMeInNow.com
http://www.AppliedMindSciences.com
http://www.AppliedWebInfo.com
http://www.BookbuilderPLUS.com
http://www.BookJumping.com
http://www.EmailNations.com
http://www.EmbarrassingProblemsFix.com
http://www.ePubWealth.com
http://www.ForensicsNation.com
http://www.ForensicsNationStore.com
http://www.FreebiesNation.com
http://www.HealthFitnessWellnessNation.com
http://www.Neternatives.com
http://www.PrivacyNations.com
http://www.RetireWithoutMoney.org
http://www.SurvivalNations.com
http://www.TheBentonKitchen.com
http://www.Theolegions.org
http://www.VideoBookbuilder.com